The Gym Life

Book of Fitness

How To Develop Full-Body Fitness That Makes You Look, Feel and Perform Better At Everything!

By Colin Stuckert

AGymLife.com

Contents

Welcome to the Gym Life Book of Fitness

In the following pages, I'm going to teach you how to develop elite fitness by taking an intelligent, balanced and health-conscious approach to training. This will include protocols for improving your strength, flexibility, movement, rest and recovery, sports, and play. My goal with this book is for you to learn how to, safely and efficiently, develop full-body, **general fitness**.

When you increase your fitness, you become better at everything. This is known as General Physical Preparedness—GPP for short—and it not only makes you more efficient at performing physical tasks, but it is also the best way of injury-proofing your body.

Increasing your GPP allows you to progress towards all of the fitness and sports-specific goals you are training towards. GPP prepares you for the "unknown." This is the kind of balanced and well-rounded fitness that military, police and fire fighters must develop because they never know what physical challenge they will face. For them, weakness in any one area—like climbing a fence or obstacle or in/out of a window—could result in serious injury or death.

Developing general fitness also makes men look "ripped" and women "lean and tone." Look at the actors from the movie 300 and you'll get the idea. Because of the balanced, full-body nature of general fitness, training for it results in a "natural" look instead of the "big" or "bulky" look (which you get from isolation exercises). Developing general fitness is not a protocol for gaining size or mass, it develops the human form to be lean, slim, and fit. (If your goal is to get big, you will have to add specific training in addition to your general fitness work.)

The protocols in this book will help you get the "fit" and "functional" look that not only looks great in the mirror but also serves as the most functional tool you will ever own. There is no fluff or long-winded science that gets in the way—only actionable protocols for building world-class fitness. (There are resources at the end of the book should you decide to pursue further study into these topics.)

After you develop a solid plan for developing your fitness, you can focus on specific goals to your hearts content. But remember: this is a book of fitness. My goal with these pages is to teach you how to build balanced fitness, and to make you want to do so. Think of the protocols of this book as the "foundation" of your fitness. Then, add goal-specific training on top of this foundation and you have a full-body, life-changing system for getting you to exactly where you want to be.

If you have any questions or comments, please shoot me an email: ismynamecolin@gmail.com. I'm here to help anyway I can.

Your body is a tool and a weapon. Let's sharpen it to a fine edge.

Yours in Fitness,

-Colin Stuckert

P.S. Make sure you get all the free Gym Life guides at www.GymLifeClub.com

Fundamentals of Fitness

The Fitness Industry

I've been coach for five years. After stumbling on HIIT training after clicking on tiny link at the end of an article on MensHealth.com (at the time, I was following a typical bodybuilding protocol), I fell into a deep hole of obsessive research. HIIT-style training opened my mind to the idea of "quantifiable fitness," and the fact that there were many ways to train the body other than just using machines and dumbbells. So I scoured the Internet, forums, articles, videos, and books on all things fitness and results-getting. As I became more and more obsessed with my results, I was constantly testing new protocols in an attempt to get them faster. To say the least, I've tried many protocols most of which didn't work or weren't effective enough to be worth my time. The recommendations in this book are based on the protocols that worked and that I use to this day.

Throughout my pursuit of knowledge in all things fitness and health, I turned to the top experts in various fields to learn from (Kelly Starrett and Mark Rippetoe as examples) and you should do the same. If you want to further pursue the study and research side of the topics in this book, start with the top coaches and authors and avoid the majority of the mainstream stuff.

In this book, I'm going to provide only simple to understand guidelines so you can get taking action immediately. I'm purposefully not going to cite studies or research; this is a book about implementation. The protocols you are going to learn work. They work for me and have worked for hundreds of clients that have trained at my box, The Training Box. They also work for the many hundreds of thousands athletes around the world that use similar methods.

That said, it's still up to you to develop the "program" that works best for you. You do this by testing and tweaking. By analyzing the results you get from the protocols you implement, you'll figure out what your body responds to best. The more you do this, the closer you'll get to your perfect program. Your perfect program will look different than mine or anyone else's. This process will take time, so be patient, keep an open mind and be ready for the long run.

Get Doing...

My expertise lies in getting people better: stronger, fitter and healthier. I've trained hundreds of clients at The Training Box since we opened in 2009. This experience has taught me a lot about training, results, and people. I've also learned the secret to getting results... and I'm going to share it with you here, right now. It's this:

Consistently showing up to do the work is the most important thing.

And...

Most people, as in 95% of the people I've seen go through the process, can't do this.

I've seen people get life-changing results after a few months of dedicated effort only to squander it soon after because they "got busy" (or some other excuse). Sure, I may be a bit jaded after seeing so many people give up like this, but after so many years and so many people, I've come to learn and accept this as a fact. (And it's one of the reasons I feel so compelled to write.)

There are oodles of health and fitness information floating around the universe. You can go to Google right now and type in anything relating to fitness and get a few million results in less than a second. The thing is, 99.99% of those results will be bias, misinformed, to downright lies most of which are meant to sell you some crap product you don't need. For whatever reason, the health and fitness industries have always attracted the charlatans and snake-oil-salesmen-types that love to tout the newest supplement, protein bar or "secret" program that'll supposedly get you results. This has leads to a public that is confused and largely misinformed.

> "Whenever you find yourself on the side of the majority, it is time to pause and reflect."
>
> -Mark Twain

As far as fitness goes, anything you hear as "common knowledge" is always inaccurate in someway. What your "fit" friend tells you is likely out of context, even if offered with the best intentions. What the trainer at the gym tells you is probably misguided, not the full story, or meant to sell you expensive personal training. What you hear and see on TV is almost always pure crap you should immediately forget.

Now, I know what you are thinking, "What makes you different?" Well, you are wise to ask this question, and actually, I'm glad you did. I want this to be your new mindset: **question everything**. Seek answers by doing your own research testing.

No, I'm not deflecting.

I'll tell you what makes me different. It's this: I share only what has worked for me, and what I've seen work, first hand, for others. See, I have this bad habit called honesty. It's far too difficult for me to write something that is made up or contrived. In fact, I have a hard time writing about anything I don't already know well (research papers destroyed me in school).

The protocols in this book are based on what I believe will work for you because they have worked for others and myself.

And still, I want you to test them out for yourself. No program or recommendation in the world will works for everyone. Sometimes you need to make subtle changes. Everyone has their own level of fitness, their own weaknesses, and their own amount of volume they will need to train safely and effectively.

Also, I recommend you check out AGymLife.com to find more of my work (and the social proof there) to help you feel more comfortable following my recommendations. That said, your job is still the same: **do the work and figure it out for yourself**.

To test new protocols for yourself:

1. Implement a recommendation
2. Gauge your results after 30 days
3. Make subtle changes for the next go-round
4. Go for another 30 days
5. Reevaluate and repeat

You should follow the above procedure with each recommendation in this book. Choose one or two protocols and incorporate them into your routine as is. Make subtle tweaks if they make sense to you (keyword: subtle). After a month of two, evaluate your results. If you are getting results, keep going. If you are struggling with results, evaluate how strict you have been and if your lifestyle factors need work (nutrition, sleep, stress). Then make the appropriate changes and get back to work. Repeat this cycle until you have built your perfect program.

This brings me to an important aspect of training that is seldom covered in popular literature. It's called belief. As with anything in life, must believe in your training efforts for them to have the best effect. Your brain is a mercurial ruler that will sabotage your best efforts if it doesn't believe—or understand—what you are doing. Even the slightest shred of doubt can cause problems. This is partly why I encourage you to make subtle tweaks when building your program because it will make you feel like it's <u>your program</u>. When you believe in your program, your brain will be your greatest ally instead of your worst enemy.

Are You Ready To Buy What I'm Selling?

I'm here to sell you two things. The first is **results**. You will get them, and it's going to be awesome. The second thing I am selling you is **hard work**. The thing is, these two come as a packaged deal—you can't have one without the other. They are exactly equal.

If you work the principles in this book—plus clean eating—you will get life changing results. I promise you that. The thing is, these results are on the other side of the mountain that is hard work, rest and nutrition. And this mountain is going to shallow you up the second you wavier in your commitment to crossing it.

I'm going to give you the protocols that work. They work for me and have worked for hundreds of clients (plus millions around the world that use similar principles). I'm not going to go into the theory and science beyond simple explanation; we have better things to do… like train.

The only thing that matters is hard work.
The only thing that matters is hard work.
The only thing that matters is hard work.

Have I emphasized this point enough? Ok, good… moving on.

The Basics of Fitness

No matter what your preferred flavor of training is, whether it is bodybuilding, gymnastics, dance, weightlifting, swimming, endurance, or picking up rocks in the forest, the only thing that is going to produce results for you is **gut-wrenching-hard-work**.

If you aren't ready to do hard work, you have no chance in hell. When you do anything physical (or in life) you should do it to the best of your ability and as hard as you can. This is where your results are hidden: beyond comfort, beyond the easy way, and beyond what most are willing to do.

Your workouts should scare you. If you are going to do bicep curls (we know you will), then you should at least do them as hard as you can. There should be intensity. You should grunt and struggle through the effort. If you are going to run a mile, you should book it as hard as you can until you can't take another step. If you are going to snatch, snatch aggressively and slam your feet into the ground as you stick the catch. If you are going to do push-ups, do them fast, hard and with concentrated effort (and no "worming").

The universal law of training that each human must abide by is: you must struggle through the effort. If your training is "easy going," "comfortable" or "moderately-paced," then you aren't training hard enough and your lack of results will show it.

Always think: I'm going to work harder than the next guy. Create an imaginary opponent in your mind. Now, every time you train, visualize his punk-ass in front of you looking back with a mocking grin. Crush him.

So now that we got the motivational stuff out of the way, and hopefully you understand what it's going to take, let's get to the doing.

Fitness, Strength and Wellness

Fundamental #1: Lift Heavy Things

Humans are made to pick up heavy things. We all need to regularly engage this stimulus to develop global fitness, increase bone density and strength, and to "bulletproof" our body as best as possible from trauma and disease. There is no shortcut or way around this. To be a fit and healthy human being requires resistance training that pushes the limits of an individual's muscular ability. Neglecting this aspect of your fitness is… well… death. Without muscular stimuli, your body will breakdown, or in other words: you will start to die. Harsh? Not in the slightest. This is just science, folks. (Study)

Women: Contrary to popular misbelief, lifting heavy weights won't make you bigger, it'll make you toner and firmer. The amount of work—and hormones—required to build muscle is of epic proportions, and even the majority of guys struggle with it. It's as if certain (not all) females think that merely touching a barbell will grow large, bulky muscles. Well as much as I wish this were the case, it couldn't be further from the truth.

The biological fact of this matter is this: As a female, you don't have the genetic make-up to get "big." For men and women alike, getting "big" or "bulky" is the result of eating lots of calories, training a ton of volume, and/or taking drugs. For females that just want to look "firm" and "tone," lifting weights is the single best thing you can do to get there.

Nutrition is the most determining factor in the size of a human, and women are no different. If you are worried about getting "big" from lifting weights then you should watch what you eat, not what you lift.

Guys: If you want to get "bigger," you need to eat plenty of calories from clean starches, proteins and fat (probably quadruple the amount of fat and protein you are eating now).

Guys or Gals: If you want to gain mass while lifting weights, do this:

1. Eat 1-2 grams of protein per pound of bodyweight per day.
2. Eat lots of clean fat (I'm talking scoopfuls).
3. Eat lots of veggies and starch (potatoes, yams, squash, white rice).

Guys or Gals: If you want to lose fat and/or maintain a healthy weight while lifting weights, do this:

1. Eat a handful size serving of protein each meal.
2. Keep meals to 2-3 times a day. Don't snack.
3. Eat clean calories from a Paleo/Primal based diet.
4. Avoid dairy, calorie-loaded drinks and anything processed.

Fundamental #2: Conditioning and Play

The 2ⁿᵈ part of the fitness and health paradigm is what most people refer to as "cardio." I prefer the definition known as metabolic conditioning. Your body has 3 metabolic pathways, or energy systems, for fueling performance. These are known as the phosphagen pathway, the glycolytic pathway, and the oxidative pathway. The phosphagen pathway powers high-power activities lasting less than 10 seconds (think weightlifting). The glycolytic pathway powers medium-powered activities lasting up to several minutes (think intervals). The third pathway, the oxidative energy system, controls low-powered activity lasting more than several minutes (endurance).

Every physical act you perform falls within one or more of these pathways. The fundamental goal of exercise is to train in these pathways so you become better adapted at performing in them. For the pursuit of general fitness, you want to avoid training too much in one pathway to the neglect of the others—like training only endurance (oxidative) and never sprinting (which targets the other two pathways).

By sufficiently training each metabolic pathway, you will develop balanced, global fitness. In a nutshell, this is how you "get fit." It's how you develop the ripped and functional look like the actors from 300.

Don't Specialize. Generalize.

It's time to start thinking of your fitness as more than a program, routine, or brand. Fitness is the culmination, and balance, of many things. The more you specialize in one modality, the more you neglect something else. While I'm not saying specialization is bad, you still have to make sure you are cognizant of the pros and cons of everything you are doing. Remember, it's all a balance.

After you have a solid foundation of fitness that targets the three pathways over various modalities, you can focus on specific training for your goal or sport—like long-distance running/cycling, sprinting, gymnastics, Olympic weightlifting, climbing, etc.

The recommendations I'm going to provide in the following pages are targeted at general fitness. Specialized training should be done with an experienced coach in addition to your general fitness program. The foundations for developing general fitness are the same whether you are a professional athlete or a soccer mom just looking to get in shape. The basics of fitness are always: lift heavy things, train the metabolic pathways, and maintain the human body through recovery, nutrition and lifestyle.

A template for developing general fitness that I have had the most success with is:

1. Train long distance at least once a week. (Row, Run, Swim, Sport, Hike, Jog)
2. Weightlifting/resistance training 2-3 times a week. (Compound lifts, functional accessory movements, and gymnastics)
3. Do something physical outdoors two or more times per week. (Sports, hike, run a hill, walking, playing)
4. Short, high-powered interval training 2-3 times a week— usually after strength sessions. (WODS, sprints, intervals, Tabata)
5. Skill and accessory work during warm-up and cool downs and on active rest days.

This template can be modified depending on your fitness level and goals, but overall this is what your average training week should look like for developing general fitness. If you are new to fitness, you'll probably need more rest days (and don't skimp on your nutrition and sleep). If you've been a "gym warrior" for years now, your volume and intensity will have to be adjusted to take that into consideration (and you'll more likely benefit the outside of the gym protocols). Regardless of your goals or current fitness level, you'll have to experiment with the dose until you find what your baseline is that you can then build on.

Fundamental #3: Maintain Nutrition, Stress, Mindset, and Lifestyle

This category includes everything else in your life that supports (or detracts from) your training efforts. The ironic thing for most people here is the effort they put into this category is likely to produce far greater results than the first two categories combined. Simply put: lifestyle is huge for your results. The big three in the lifestyle category are food, sleep and stress. Sleep is simple: get more of it. Stress is a huge topic beyond the scope of this book. A quick recommendation for mitigating stress is to look into the following: meditation, mindfulness, and philosophy (Stoicism is my favorite). Then we have nutrition.

Many experts (I think Mark Sisson also says this) believe that food comprises 80% or more of your body composition and long-term health. My personal opinion—from what I've seen over and over again—is it's at least that. Really, regardless of what percentage it is for you, the fact remains: <u>If you aren't prepared to work on your nutrition, you are severely handicapping your health and results</u>.

If there were only one thing you could take away from this book it would be this:

<u>**If you want to live an amazing life, with a body that looks good and is free of disease and medical complication, then you must eat right, exercise and maintain a healthy lifestyle.**</u>

Ok, but what if you don't care about being healthy? Well, I think you are crazy, but do you at least care about your results? Do you care what you look like in the mirror? <u>If so,</u>

then you should want to invest effort into the lifestyle category because they are what determine how your body looks.

Exercise is only a smidgen of the pie that represents your body and health… a smidgen.

Besides, health is sexy, and the more you do to promote your health, the faster your results will come (a double whammy of sexiness). If you combine lifestyle protocols with hard work on your fitness, you'll crush your goals in no time. In fact, you'll have to set new goals because the old ones will soon be outdated. Have I convinced you yet? I hope so because a life—which is determined by your health—is a terrible thing to waste.

Let's review the three fundamentals of fitness:

Fundamental #1: Lift Heavy Things
Fundamental #2: Get Moving: Conditioning, Cardio, Metabolic, Play
Fundamental #3: Maintain your life: Nutrition, Sleep, Stress, Mindset, Mobility, Balance

The Numbers

Before we get to the nitty-gritty action-taking protocols that are going to be responsible for turning your body into the statue of David, or Aphrodite for the ladies, I first must share an unpleasant truth with you. The truth to all this fitness and goal-stuff is: the majority of people never reach their goals.

The statistics show that most of you reading this won't make it. There are many reasons why this is so. You'll wax and wane, yo-yo, and struggle to develop the habits you need to stick with it. This could go on for months, even years, until you reach the tipping point and either solidify the habit or quit for good. As unfortunate as this is, it's reality. We must face the truth. I tell you this to prepare you. Yes, you should be a little scared with all this. A little bit of fear is good for keeping you only our toes. Take this stuff seriously... it's your freaking life.

Now, **you** have a much better chance than others to not end up another statistic because you have me to give it to you straight and point you in the right direction. And to kick-off this partnership in getting you fit, I need you to do something. I want you to, right now, make a commitment to yourself that you are going to stick with your program. Say it out loud. Write it down. Tape it to your mirror and fridge. Put a note in your car. Send yourself automated Google calendar email reminders (I do all of these). Something like this will work:

I commit to building the habits of health and fitness. This will include getting enough sleep, eating clean, natural foods, training hard multiple days a week, and taking time off to relax and small the roses.

Now, my commitment to you:

I'm going to do everything I can to help you get there. If you get stuck or have questions, send me an email and I will get back to you. ismynamecolin@gmail.com

Your best offense against failure is your brain. The more you understand this process, the easier it is to do the work. The more you believe in what you are doing, the easier it is to do the work. The more educated you are about all this, the easier it is to do the work. The more resilient you are mentally, the easier it is to do the work. Train your mind and you train your body. Remember, I'm here to help. Let's do work.

Results-getting is easy(ier) when you have the right information.

You now have a leg-up on everyone else because you have the following guidelines—void of fluff, filler, or bias—that are going to teach you the fundamentals of fitness. You also have access to the Internet and the limitless resources that show you how to squat, eat, cook, and so on (some of which: www.GymLifeClub.com and www.GymLifeCook.com).

Let's Talk About Habits

It's obscenely difficult to make or break habits. Doing either requires you to fight your brain's desire to take the path of least resistance. Habits are the source of everything in your life good or bad. When you achieve success, thank your habits. When you fail, thank your habits. The reason people don't reach their goals is because they quit long before developing the habits. This is what the numbers say will be true for you: you will give up (and that is why you will fail).

Make a commitment to yourself to not let this happen.

As you start on this journey, should you feel yourself waning in your commitment, do something drastic to relight the fire. Do anything; be creative. Write 100 memo notes and post them around your house. Set timers, calendar reminders, email reminders. Call a friend and ask them to keep you—or each other—accountable with regular check-ins. Hang your workout clothes on your front door handle. And so on.

Habit research shows that small acts are the key to big acts because the small acts initiate the big acts. These are called "triggers" because they subconsciously start the process in your mind that leads you to the bigger effort. Use triggers to get yourself to start when you aren't motivated to.

Further reading: http://zenhabits.net/triggers-and-habits/

The Self of You

There is a war raging on and you are smack-dab in the middle. This war is fought between two armies vying for dominance on the battlefield between your ears. From now until the end of your life, you are going to be stuck in the middle of a war between these opposing parts of your self.

We all wax and wane in life. Sometimes our motivation is high, sometimes it is low. Sometimes we are on a good streak, sometimes we aren't. This is an expression of the war that is ranging on inside you head between taking and not taking action. It's having an angel and devil on each shoulder. Let's see how this battle affects your exercise habits.

The devil wants you to skip the gym and buy a tub of ice cream on your way home from work so you can watch American Idol while stuffing your face with sugar. The angel wants you to go the gym and exercise so you will relieve stress from work and feel good about making a healthy decision. The angel is the general of your "Motivated" army that represents all the healthy, goal-inducing habits. The devil is in command of army "Lazy" which is composed of in-action, laziness, sloth, and the other unhealthy habits that take you further away from your goals.

For most people, the Lazy army has more troops than the Motivated army (most of us have society and our coddled upbringing to blame for this). Because you are reading this book I'm going to assume that you want the Angel on your shoulder to prevail. To make this happen, you must actively recruit soldiers into the Motivated army by doing things that will strengthen your resolve—like reading books and articles, listening to podcasts, meditating, practicing mindfulness, eating better, learning how to cook, going for a walk, sleeping more, etc. The more you invest in these healthy habits, the more the Motivated army grows. In time, the Motivated army will conquer the Lazy army and take control over the realm to rule in peace and harmony.

However, as any ruler knows, peace is never a lasting guarantee. Because of this, you must keep your army motivated, trained and constantly growing stronger. The more troops you have under your command, the more protection you have against the evil forces of Lazy that plot to overthrow your rule at the slightest sign of weakness.

So, if you take away anything at all from this book (and from that analogy that was really fun to write), it should be this: habits are everything.

Failure is what? (Not what you think)

Let's be clear about one thing: I don't believe in the word failure, <u>and neither should you</u>. When I say, "Many of you will fail," I really mean that many of you will give up. You will stop and revert to old ways. You will let Lazy overtake and rule the Iron Throne. Failure is a choice: it's you making the choice to quit. But the fact that failure is a choice is a very good thing.

Why is this good, you ask? Because it makes it simple: if you refuse to quit, you don't fail. As long as you keep going, you get there. Sure, you will have temporary setbacks, that's to be expected. In fact, setback is just another word for failure... if you give up. If you don't quit, then a setback is just a temporary lull. See how that works?

Your results may not come as fast as you'd like, but if you keep going, nothing can stand in your way. This process is a journey. As I sit here and write these words in an attempt to help you along this path, I still struggle with aspects of my health and fitness. Some weeks I eat better than others (don't ask me about last week), and some days I have more energy to train while other days I feel like a complete weakling-newbie. It's all part of the journey. But what separates me from most is I never quit. I've been training for 12 years and the longest I've ever gone without stepping foot in a gym was 30 days (I had some tragic "life stuff" I was dealing with at the time).

It's hard, not impossible

There are many bear traps lying in the weeds waiting to foil your journey to Results Land. These traps want to keep you fat, sick, and plugged into the matrix as a blind consumer. The only way to combat these dangers is to develop your mindset, your Angel army of Motivated warriors called habits. You do this through education (like this) and consistent action-taking.

Back To The Mind

Training your mindset—and the belief system—is just as important as training your body (more important for those of you that have a massive Lazy army calling the shots). Think about it: mindset is the root to all your decision-making and action-taking. Get it right or you have no chance in hell of battling the evil, dark forces of Lazy.

Your mindset is the most important thing in <u>your</u> universe.

I think I've covered enough of the intangibles for getting results. It's now time we move to the doing. But before we do, I must remind you that the knowledge you gain relating to fitness (or anything) will translate to diddly squat if you don't put in the work. Again I will remind you: the number one reason people fail to get results is they don't stay consistent—they give up. (It's funny cuz in person I hate repeating myself, and rarely do it. Shows you how serious something is when I say it more than once.)

The Fitness Template
(printable version in resources section)

1. Weightlifting: Lift weights 2-4 times a week. Focus on the big lifts: Deadlift, Squat, Bench Press, Press, Clean, Jerk, Snatch. Use functional accessory movements to compliment these lifts: Pull-ups, Dips, Push-ups, Pistols, One-arm PU/PU, Plyometrics, Kettlebell Swings, etc.

2. Conditioning: Sprint, Carry, Lift, Drag and Throw, Run Long Distance Sometimes, Row, Swim, Bike, Play Sports, Skip the elliptical, and Forget The Treadmill (go outside).

3. Follow a program, listen to your body and train it hard: Follow a weightlifting program and a GPP program as your foundation of general fitness. A general GPP program can do wonders for developing fitness. After you have your base, add goal-specific training.

4. Rest intelligently: Most of you will need at least two full days of rest a week, some will need more. If you hate rest—like many of us do—you can spend time with active recovery in the form of yoga, walking, hiking, and other low-intensity physical activity.

5. Eat a clean diet: The bulk of your calories should come from the highest-quality protein and fat you can find. Eat fewer carbs on your rest days and a bit more on training days in the form of starchy veggies and sweet potatoes. High-volume trainees should regulate carb levels to support performance (test and tweak).

6. Manage lifestyle factors: Sleep, stress, recovery, etc.

There you have it, the basics for making all your body dreams come true. If you focus on these fundamentals, you have the power to build the body and health you deserve. Don't complicate it. Don't let a lack of understanding hold you back.

You don't need to understand WHY these protocols work, they do, so get doing. (And if you want to know more, see the Resources section at the end of the book.)

If you take the six steps listed above, and put in work for each one—especially diet and lifestyle—you'll see massive, life changing results. That is my guarantee. You know what you need to do. It's now time to get to the doing. If you need help along the way, please email me: ismynamecolin@gmail.com. Get all of my future updates and the Gym Life bonuses at www.GymLifeClub.com.

Lift Heavy Things

I remember watching a video of Dave Tate—powerlifting legend and owner of EliteFTS—as he explained the importance of increasing strength. He said, "Increasing maximal strength increases everything else [of your fitness] at the same time."

He's so very right.

Developing strength increases your proficiency in every other marker of health and fitness, and should a forefront goal for everyone (men, women, big, small, old, young). Building muscle mass makes the human figure look fit, slim, and sexy. It also makes a human being more likely to live long and prosper.

Building muscle mass is the best way to "bulletproof" your body and ward off disease. Strength can save your life should you find yourself in a life-threatening situation. No matter how you spin it, strength is pretty freaking awesome and necessary. If you haven't already, it's time you implement a program for developing strength.

Lifting Weights and Size

Contrary to popular (mis)belief, lifting weights does not just make you "big." Sure, there are exceptions to this, but for 99% of men and women (maybe 99.9999% for women) getting "big," "huge," or "jacked" is not a realistic expectation from lifting weights alone. Calories, drugs, and supplements—and lots and lots of training—are what determines the amount of size a human develops from resistance training.

*For the females reading, know this: It takes us guys a massive amount of effort in many categories—plus favorable genetics—to get "big." For you, you need not worry about getting big from resistance training. Plus, you can always STOP lifting weights if you started seeing your body getting bigger in the mirror, could you not? Muscle takes months, even years, to grow. You won't wake up tomorrow with huge quads because you did a few sets of squats the day before (I wish it was that easy). Weights will help you tone, firm, and build the body you want as a woman. This cannot be said of running, the elliptical, ab exercises, leg raises, or dance class—it's best to treat these as accessories to your resistance training).

"Strong people are harder to kill and more useful in general."

-Mark Rippetoe

Size vs. strength

A point I want to clarify before we move on is the difference between size (being "big") and strength (the skill of moving weight). In a nutshell, big does not always equal strong and strong does not always equal big. Let's consider the male gymnast as an example. Did you know that gymnasts are the strongest, pound-for-pound, athletes in the world relative to their bodyweight? Most people wouldn't consider gymnasts "big" or think of one when referring to the "strongest athlete," but such is the case. Gymnasts are strong and not big because the focus of their training is bodyweight based, which is based on training relative loads (bodyweight) and not external, maximal loads (external weights).

On the other end of the strength spectrum, let's look to the sport of strongman, which produces athletes that are big and strong. Strongmen are required to move external loads (weight) instead of relative loads like the gymnast. This is the fundamental difference in strength application—between maximal and relative—that I want you to understand as it correlates to the size of muscle as well as strength development.

Because the goal of strongman is to move as much weight as possible, being big and strong are fundamental to the sport. More muscle surface area, or muscle mass, provides more room for muscle to develop condensed muscle fibers that are necessary to move massive external loads. Strongmen are big and strong because they aim to move the greatest amount of external weight as possible, and their training and body-type reflect such.

Another sport that can help showcase the difference between size and strength—and highlight a bit of a paradox when it comes to the two—is the sport of powerlifting. The goal of powerlifting is to lift the most amount of weight possible in three movements: bench, squat and deadlift. For the heaviest weight classes, powerlifters are usually "bigger" because, like strongmen, their goal is to move the most weight possible, and they need as much muscle mass as possible to achieve that goal.

As you move down in weight classes among powerlifters—and where we find what seems like a paradox—we find athletes at the lower classes that look like regular "everyday" people yet posses the strength to move large amounts of external loads relative to their bodyweight. Many of these athletes wouldn't be considered "big" at all by most people's standards. To explain why this is within the sport of powerlifting, and how it applies to highlighting the difference between size and strength, we look to the weight classes themselves.

Since all athletes under 264 pounds (198 pounds for women), which represent the heaviest weight classes, fall into partitioned weight classes, controlling ones size and weight is necessary to staying within in a specific class. In this instance, it would be counterproductive to put on too much size as that could move an athlete into a higher weight class where he or she could be outmatched by heaver, and stronger, competition. The difference here is the heaviest weight classes for men and women have no cap on the weight of athletes. Athletes must be a minimum of weight for the weight class and can become as big and heavy as so desired. In this case, there would be no determent to adding more size if it allowed an athlete to move more weight.

All sports have different modalities and goals indicative to the sport, and each produces a body-type best suited for optimal performance in that sport. The sport of gymnastics is centered on body control, which requires athletes to develop large amounts of joint and ligament strength as needed to perform complex body movements and holds. The strength required for this modality is different from the strength required by a powerlifter or strongman that must move as much external weight as possible.

The last example we will look at is the sport of Bodybuilding. Bodybuilder's primary training goal is ascetics—size and proportion. Strength is not a factor in bodybuilding competitions at all. This is why bodybuilders focus on training for hypertrophy, or the size of a muscle, in combination with balance and symmetry. Hypertrophy is best developed using relatively light weights compared to what powerlifters and strongmen use in pursuing of strength (which again showcases the paradox between size and strength).

The lesson here is this: The size of muscle does not always correlate to strength because there is a difference between training for strength, which also includes developing the central nervous system (CNS), and training for size, which is the result of inducing micro tears that lead to growing a muscle larger. There are also a difference in the amount of condensed muscle fibers of a muscle that is independent of size. As a general rule, smaller athletes that are strong relative to their size because they train primarily strength protocols will have more condensed muscle fibers while larger athletes that train primarily for size are likely to have less condensed muscle fibers.

In summary, size does not equal strength and strength does not equal size. Each are independent variables with their own set of rules and best practices for developing.

Here is a Simplified view of the various differences between training for size and strength (of course, there is overlap between all of these):

Body Control and relative strength: The primary focus of the gymnast, which includes bodyweight movements, balancing and static holds. Conditioning is done using bodyweight exercises, plyometrics, static holds for time, and movement-based skill work. This method of training primarily develops strength and movement skills and is not ideal for producing muscle size.

Maximal Strength: The strength sought by powerlifters and strongmen with the goal of moving the most external weight possible. Size and strength can be developed using these methods, but strength is the primary pursuit. Training primarily consists of moving heavy weights in the 70% (of 1RM) zones in the form of complex, functional lifts like the deadlift, squat, bench press, press, clean, jerk, row, sled-pulls, tire flips, and farmer carries.

Hypertrophy or the size of a muscle: The primary goal of bodybuilding, hypertrophy is trained using lots of reps at lighter weights and strategic rest periods for allowing the micro tears in muscles to grow larger. Hypertrophy methods are best for producing the size of a muscle and not necessarily it's strength. Features include plenty of reps with as much TUT (time under tension) as possible while utilizing "isolation" exercises at light to medium weights.

In summary, if you want size, you must train and eat for it. If you want strength and want to minimize size, you should train for it and adjust your calories to support that goal. If you want strength and size, you must train for it, eat for it and adjust the many external factors necessary based on your genetic makeup. And at the end of the day, your genetics and nutrition are going to play the largest role in how your body develops.

Muscle size is the combination of training, nutrition and lifestyle habits. If you adjust these factors to produce size— whether accidentally or on purpose—you will produce size to the point that your genetic capabilities allow. If you adjust these factors to be lean and ripped, you will produce leanness and ripped-ness. Because we all posses different genetics, it will come down to a ton of testing and tweaking to figure out what works best for you.

And, no matter what, strength should be a focused pursuit!

Whether you want to get big, small, tone, or lean, you will get closer to your goals by taking a strength-first approach. If you focus on strength and add in hypertrophy training, you'll get more size than from training only strength protocols. If you only want strength and not size, then I recommend you focus on the three basic lifts—squat, deadlift, press—in conjunction with plenty of bodyweight conditioning, sprinting and HIIT-focused conditioning (and a clean diet).

Some of these concepts might seem obvious or redundant, and you would be right in thinking so. The thing is, most people try to do too much and make it far more complicated than it needs to be. And the more they do this, the less likely they are to get the results they are after. That is why I need to be blatantly clear with the principles that get you results. Stick to the fundamentals... where your results are waiting for you.

"It's not the daily increase but daily decrease. Hack away at the unessential."

"Simplicity is the key to brilliance."

-Bruce Lee

A Template For Strength and Fitness

The following template is what I recommend as the baseline for everyone. It will develop foundational and balanced strength and full-body fitness. For most of you, this is a great place to start. For those of you that are advanced, you can use this as a foundation to build on as you will still need to develop balanced general fitness.

The Baseline:

For strength sessions, lift a mix of heavy, medium and light weights as many reps and sets needed to reach failure. Go to failure most of the time, near failure sometimes and just short of failure the rest of the time. Stick with 2-4 lifting days a week (three is the sweet spot). Incorporate conditioning and play throughout the week between weight sessions. Utilize active rest days. Get a ton of sleep. Eat a clean diet with lots of protein and fat.

Remember, everyone is different and responds differently to training. For your specific genetics and level of fitness, you may require more or less volume.

*To build strength: Lift heavy weights in the 70%+ range (of your 1 rep max) in the 3-7 rep ranges for 3-5 sets. Increase weights and volume as you get stronger. Take a deload week every two months or so. Train 4 days a week and let your body rest the other days (and use active rest). Check out Jim Wendler's 5/3/1 program for a simple and effective strength program to follow.

*To build size: Lift light, medium, and heavy weights using lots of reps and sets. Utilize hypertrophy-based exercises. My favorites are: Weighted Pull-up, Dip, Squat, Deadlift, Front Squat, Press, and Bench. Eat a lot of clean calories and plenty of carbs in the form of white rice, sweet potatoes and starchy veggies.

Follow a Program

The key to training success is consistency. Within the confines of a consistent program, you will have a balance of light days, rest days, heavy days, and in-between days. No one can train at their highest level year-round. Athletes have an off-season for a reason. Your body will tell you what it can handle if you listen to it and scale up or down based on the feedback you get.

I recommend everyone follow program because it makes training easier and keeps you accountable. For strength, stick to one of these tested and true classics: Starting Strength by Mark Rippetoe or 5/3/1 by Jim Wendler. These programs can be used by beginners as well as advanced athletes. The difference will lie in the numbers. Getting bigger and stronger, even at the highest levels, requires a linear increase of weight and reps to elicit the proper hormonal and muscular response to bring about growth and development. This is basic human biology. The strongest guys and gals in the world still squat, deadlift, and move like the rest of us—they just do it more, heavier, better and faster.

Each Workout:

1) Body Temp Warm-up: Jog, Row, and move for 5 minutes until you break a sweat.
2) Dynamic Warm-up: Use movement-based exercises to loosen joints and prime motor pathways.
3) Strength: Perform one or two main lifts a day to failure or near-failure. Follow a program.
4) Accessory Exercises: Add 2-5 complimentary exercises to each main lift and perform 8-15 reps over 3-5 sets. For example, do single-leg squats, weighted lunges and glute-ham raises on your squat day, and dips, floor presses and clapping push-ups on your chest/shoulder day.

5) Conditioning: Complete 5-25 minutes of high-intensity conditioning work.

6) Cool-down: Stretch, jog, walk, and keep moving for 5 minutes to let your body cool down gradually.

Above is the basic template for your in-the-gym training days. Mix up the conditioning aspect of your workouts often. The days you aren't "feeling" your conditioning, skip it. If your body is sore and weak but you still want to do something, use an active rest days. The same goes for your strength training. If you feel strong, do more volume. If you feel weak, consider an off day. No program, coach, or Internet forum in the world can tell you what your body is telling you. Listen to it.

That's it. It's not complicated. **It just takes consistency and hard work**. Follow this template 2-4 times a week, while coupled with a clean, Paleo-based diet, and you will produce life-changing results.

Remember, the most important thing is showing up consistently. So make sure you...

...get the work done no matter what!

Don't complicate it. Grab a program, plug in your numbers, and get working. Then follow it up with proper nutrition, sleep, and recovery.

Training Tips:

Warm-up to your heavy sets slowly. Don't just slap 225 on the bar and start squatting. That is how you hurt yourself.

Rest 1-2 minutes between sets. Watch the clock—take your rest intervals seriously.

Mix up the amount of weight you lift and the reps and sets from time to time.

Follow a program.

Train hard with perfect form.

Utilize spotters when going heavy.

Train with someone. You will train harder and it will show in your results. Plus, it's safer.

Foam roll before training.

Work on mobility and keep your joints healthy.

Don't overtrain. There is too much of a good thing.

Sleep 8 hours a night. Lifting heavy requires it.

Don't assume you will get big. Some of you with certain genetics might get bigger, most wont. It's usually diet and drugs that make a human "big."

Stay consistent and take a week off every couple months. It will improve your results.
Train on an empty stomach.

Protein and water post-workout will improve recovery (use a quality grass-fed protein).

If you want to get big, you have to eat big.

If you want that sexy, slim and fit look, you have to lift weights and eat clean.

Gymnastics

Building strength and flexibility through body control

I'm a fan of natural movement; from climbing, running, balancing, or crawling in the forest, to sports that utilize body control such gymnastics and break dancing, to street performers that perform amazing feats of strength and skill, to the Cirque Du Soleil shows that fill stadiums with their impressive dancers and athletes. Of it all, I'm a fan. But before we get into the specifics of this kind of training—and how it can take your results to an entirely new level, let's look at a brief history of how the sport of gymnastics came to be.

Gymnastics originated in Greece as a method of physically preparing soldiers for war (cool). The Greeks believed that the skills of gymnastics—jumping, tumbling, running, and mounting and dismounting horses—were assets on the battlefield. Since the Greeks celebrated physical fitness in men and women, gymnazein, which means, "to exercise naked," became a vital part of Greek education. This came to an unfortunate end when the Roman Empire conquered the Greeks and gymnastics fell out of favor in education to be reserved for training the military.

Training soldiers with the gymnastics-style modality has passed to many continents and nations since the time of the Greeks. In the early nineteenth century, the United States Military began incorporating gymnastics principles into solider training programs. Yet again, gymnastics fell out of favor when the evolution of machinery used in combat become the focus of training soldiers (to the determent of the soldiers in my opinion). Nowadays, only remnants of gymnastic-style training remain in the US military's training programs—push-ups, sit-ups, squats, and obstacle-based movements like crawling, climbing and jumping)

Sport

The sport of gymnastics began to develop in the late eighteenth century in Europe. Apparatuses such as the horizontal bar, parallel bars, pommel horse, balance beam and vaulting horse were developed by two physical educators named Johann Friedrich Gutsmuch and Friedrich Ludwig Jahn. Boys were taught how to perform skills on each apparatus and the sport of gymnastics was born. Gymnastics was first introduced into the Olympics in 1986. Since then, it has become a worldwide competition-based sport for boys, girls, men and women.

What can gymnastics do for you?

Did you know that the gymnasts you see on TV are some of the strongest—relative to their bodyweight—athletes in the world? The way a gymnast controls his body is a showcase of amazingly practical strength and skill. What you see on TV are skills that have taken years to develop. For the purpose of developing functional control, balance, and bodyweight-based strength, we will utilize the most basic forms of gymnastic movement.

By training these fundamental gymnastics skills, you will learn develop similar relative-to-bodyweight strength and body control that is so impressive among gymnasts. You will learn the skill of body control, which consists of moving and holding the body in various positions and angles. Your balance will increase as well as your awareness of what your body is doing as it moves through space. This awareness skill alone has many applications in sport and life.

Part of rounded general fitness is possessing then ability to move up, down, around, over and under an obstacle or terrain. For our ancestors, a proficiency in these movements would have been conducive for living in nature (as we have for millions of years), and is another reason I am a fan of bodyweight based training and movement—because it's natural.

Picture a toddler running around the living room. He can squat, roll and bend his body freely without pain or stiffness. This is how every human should be able to move, especially adults. The thing is, from a lack of proper movement, poor nutrition, sitting, and other constraints from living in an industrialized culture, we have become sedentary and atrophied. And our muscles, joints, and movement have suffered as a result.

Bodyweight movement is the key to unlocking the toddler inside us all. And being able to do so will pay dividends for not only your fitness results, but also your longevity as a human being. You and I are made to move, and a lot. Movement is one of the most neglected aspects of fitness for most people, even frequent gym-goers. You must move as much as you can and in as many ways as possible. Just running, or just rowing, or just weightlifting, is not moving. Those are confined modalities of movement that are restricted in their movement patterns and are performed in a rigid, repeatable fashion. While this is better than not moving at all, it is still not enough.

You Are Made To Move

When you don't climb, run, swim, crawl, or challenge your body in a wide variety of challenging and "unknown" ways on a regular basis, your body breaks down. The less you move, the less efficient you become as a mover and as a human. For better or worse, the "use it or lose it" maxim rules the human existence. (See Kelly Starrett's book: Becoming a Supple Leopard.)

When our ancestors lived as hunter-gatherers, they did not "lift" for the sake of lifting. Although they did lift heavy objects for various reasons like dragging a kill back to camp or for building shelters. Their constant movement in nature consisted of short bouts of intense effort followed by plenty of movement at a slow, leisurely pace. This created a human body that was functional, flexible, and strong.

Our ancestors entire existence revolved around movement.

Humans did, however, "play" for the sake of playing. This play usually involved functional human movement over uneven and unpredictable terrain. We would wrestle, race, and compete in ways only limited by our imagination. We would run, climb, balance, jump, throw, carry, drag, hike, and so on. And we were better in every way because of it.

Why move like this?

Because it could save your life someday…
Because it is the only way you can remain healthy...
Because it makes you lean, fit, and strong...
Because you are made to.

Imagine being stuck in a burning building, or worse, your family trapped? You might have to climb in and out of the 2nd story window to save them because the firemen will be too late. Would you be able to do it?

What if you find yourself in your car as it sinks to the bottom of a river? Your flexibility and body control could allow you to wiggle your way out of the window and save your life.

What if you trip and fall down a flight of stars? You fall better because of the body-awareness you posses. You'll tuck, roll and protect your head and neck, and it could save your life.

What if… what if anything? There are countless situations where being able to move your body effectively could save your life.

As a functioning human being, you should posses the control to be able to move your body up, down, around, and over anything that comes your way. Having this kind of body control will make you a fitter, and more prepared for the unknown, human being. You will be stronger mentally and physically because you will be in-tune with your body, and confident in your skills.

Your body is your weapon and having control of it is being skilled with this weapon.

The goal of pursuing gymnastic/bodyweight conditioning is to produce relative strength and body control. This modality of training is the perfect compliment to a basic weightlifting program. Benefits include improving your flexibility, balance, coordination, and movement.

When you combine bodyweight training with the strength development you get from lifting weights, you have the template for producing an amazingly functional—and beautiful—human body. In the words of Mark Rippetoe, you have become "harder to kill and more useful in general." But the key is…

…to balance both!

The right way to develop strength (or any part of your fitness) is to develop it in as many ways as possible. This means you aren't only lifting or only training bodyweight conditioning, **you do both.** Make it your aim to develop strength in as many modalities as possible: Light, Heavy, Medium, Climbing, Crawling, Carrying, Dragging, Bodyweight, Strongman, Olympic weightlifting, Gymnastics.

Back to gymnastics...

Now that we see how body control is useful, and how it might save your life someday, let's move to the how-to of adding it to your program. Bodyweight conditioning is, in my opinion, the most under-utilized and underrated form of physical exercise. For those of you already lifting weights, bodyweight conditioning is the perfect compliment.

Definition of gymnastics:

A. practice or training in exercises that develop physical strength and agility or mental capacity
a. Physical exercises designed to develop and display strength, balance, and agility, especially those performed on or with specialized apparatus.
b. The art or practice of such exercises.

If you have ever done a push-up or a bodyweight squat, you have done an exercise within the gymnastic realm. Any movement that moves the body without an external load is gymnastic in nature. A few sports that utilize gymnastic movement include:

- DANCING
- BREAK DANCING
- MARTIAL ARTS
- CHEERLEADING
- TUMBLING
- BALLET
- CLIMBING
- CIRQUE DU SOLEIL

Training

So how do we incorporate bodyweight conditioning into our program? There are two ways I recommend. The first is to use bodyweight movements as "accessories" during your weightlifting sessions. Lifting weights followed by bodyweight exercises are a match made in heaven—like peanut butter and jelly (which you shouldn't be eating). The results you will see with these complimenting modalities will blow your mind.

How: Use bodyweight accessory sets between and/or after your sets of weighted movements.

Example: After a heavy sets of squats, finish out with some high-rep pistol work.

Another example: Between bench sets, work sets of dips and muscle-ups.

Third example: Finish with handstand work after shoulder presses.

The "Incorporate More Bodyweight Conditioning Into Your Program" Template (interchange exercises):

1. **Main lift:** 5x5 Shoulder Press
2. **1st accessory set:** 3-5 sets of Handstand pushups
3. **2nd Accessory:** Ring or bar dips for 3-5 reps, adding weight each set
4. **3rd Accessory:** A dumbbell exercise such as DB push-presses or one-arm push-ups
5. **Finish**: Handstand walks to failure

This is what a standard strength session with bodyweight training added looks like. You perform one or two main lifts followed by 2-4 accessory exercises for each lift.

Bodyweight as Skill Work

The second way to incorporate bodyweight training into your program is to work gymnastics for 5-15 minutes each session during "skill work" time. This is best placed between your strength and conditioning work. Since bodyweight movements are so skill-intensive, you need to practice them often. The best way to do this is between your strength and conditioning work and on "active rest" days (or days you feel weak and skip lifting). Skill work is the perfect way to develop your movement without taxing your CNS and cutting into your recovery.

Practice Makes Awesome

When it comes to bodyweight training, know this: practice makes perfect. To improve, focus on slow, full-rep movements with perfect form. As your form improves, increase speed. Always take a "form first" approach.

Common bodyweight exercises
Use YouTube for exercise demos and train with a coach if possible.

Frog stands
Handstands (walks, presses, one arm, two arm)
Push-ups (one arm, clapping, etc.)
Dips (all kinds)
Pull-ups (strict, kips, one-arm, wide, narrow, under, over)
Muscle-ups (rings, bar, kip, strict)
Pistols (weighted, rolling, jumps)
Jumping (one leg, back, forward, front, lateral, height, over, under, etc.)
Planks
Planche practice (advanced)
Levers (front, back, tuck holds, advanced)
Glute-ham raises
GHD Sit-ups
Sit-ups
V-Ups
Skin-the-cat (bar, rings)
Supermans
Squats

If you wish to do further research and learn from some of the masters, check these guys out:

Coach Sommer: www.gymnasticbodies.com
Ido Portal: www.idoportal.com
Movnat: www.movnat.com

Don't miss out on the opportunity to capture more strength, more body control, more flexibility, more joint strength, more ligament strength, and the multitude of other benefits that come from bodyweight training. No matter your size, level of fitness or current goals, you will get better beyond belief by incorporating bodyweight training into your program.

Remember, it can save your life!

Conditioning and Play

Fitness and Play

This chapter covers the development of your metabolic conditioning (or "cardio") in its many forms: endurance training, interval training, playing sports, sprinting, WODs, hiking, walking, etc. For simplicity sake, we'll refer to all of these as "conditioning."

Conditioning comes in many modalities, methods, programs, and lengths. As far as length goes—which is of paramount importance—I recommend you train short, fast and hard most of the time, slow and long other times, and at a moderate pace the rest of the time. Some days you'll do your conditioning in the gym while other days you'll get outside and take a hike or play a sport. Mix it up often to keep your body guessing.

Your body requires many modalities to develop the balanced whole we refer to as fitness. The more you challenge and move your body, the more you improve your fitness. Since the definition of fitness is the ability to perform any physical task, it only makes sense that the more tasks you perform, the better your fitness develops. Right? Right.

The number one problem that trainees run into is a focusing on one or two modalities to the neglect of others—simply put: not enough variety in their training. When you train too much in one modality—long distance for example—you increase your proficiency in that modality while simultaneously developing weaknesses in other areas of your fitness. This can create wide gaps in your fitness. As I've said before, your body needs balance. There is no "best" way to train. There is only better or worse depending on your strengths and weaknesses. What you have to do is find what methods provide you more better and less worse, then do more of them until the scale shifts and your weaknesses become strengths.

Let's say you lift weights exclusively but never run. Being able to deadlift 500 pounds yet unable to run a respectable mile isn't balanced fitness. Having a gap this glaring in your fitness can kill you (like when the zombie apocalypse hits). When you are cognizant of maintain a balance in your, you'll will utilize to avoid these large gaps in your fitness. (There are stories of powerlifters getting winded as they walked to the lifting platform in competition. Sounds absurd, yes, but it still happens. There are also runners who have near zero muscle mass and would snap like a twig if put under any kind of strain. And so on.)

Your Fitness Program

Weightlifting and bodyweight training makes up the foundation of your strength development while balanced and varied conditioning take care of the rest of your fitness. Strength and conditioning compliment one another. The stronger you get, the better your conditioning gets. The more conditioned you get, the stronger you get from lifting weights and training bodyweight movements. It's a beautiful circle of awesomeness. (Disclaimer: this is assuming you take a strength-first pursuit and use conditioning intelligently—as in not too much. Too much conditioning can negate your strength development if you slip into overtraining.)

Too many trainees get sucked into a single training dogma. Runners like to consider themselves "runners" and will avoid lifting weights. Weightlifters want to be thought of as a "weightlifter" and so they won't run. The thing is, each athlete can benefit from each other modality. A true athlete is not closed-minded; he is not exclusionary or biased. He learns from everyone and finds a way to fit every useful style into his program. He constantly works on his weaknesses.

This needs to be you.

No matter what your goals are, or what training "school" you come from, you should strive to improve your general fitness by utilizing as many methods of fitness as possible. This will get you to your goals faster and safer and make you a balanced whole that is more likely to survive whatever life throws your way.

The Case For Fitness

Fitness can save your life: crawling out the window of a burning house, out of your flipped car that is stuck in the middle of oncoming traffic, or climbing to safety as a rabid dog or zombie or mugger chases you down. Situations where your physical fitness can improve your chances of survival are countless. If you are like most people (I hope not), you probably think:

"That'll never happen to me."

That's what everyone thinks until something does happen and they are left thinking, "shit." Answer this question: How many people die every day? The answer is 150,000. Now, contemplate how many of these deaths could have been prevented had the individuals been stronger in body and mind. My guess would be: plenty. Don't be another statistic.

Think of your family. Are you strong enough to protect them? Let's use the fire example again: Imagine your family is stuck in your house as it is engulfed in flames. Now consider their only chance of survival is you climbing up to the 2nd-story window and rescuing them with your own two hands because the fire department won't make it in time. Will you be able to save them?

Fitness is that freaking important!

The fitter survive. Herbert Spencer coined the term "Survival of the fittest" after reading Darwin's explanation of Natural Selection in his book On The Origin of Species. Darwin's theory of natural selection states that the organism most able to adapt to their environment has the best chance of surviving to reproduce and pass on their genes. As this cycle repeats itself through successive generations, the weak die out. This concept applies to human beings as much as it does animals in the Galapagos.

The "fitter" you are, the more likely you are to find a mate, reproduce, and raise offspring. Additionally, the stronger you are—mentally and physically—the better you will perform in all matters of life, not just reproduction. Want to survive the next flu pandemic? Be stronger. Want to survive should the government break down and fire, police and the paramedics are nowhere to be found? Be stronger. And the list goes on and on.

While some of you might think these are only "doomsday" scenarios, and they are, it does not make them any less able to happen. And don't forget, people die everyday even in the "safest" parts of the world. Rape, murder, disease, sickness, etc., the list goes on.

It's your genetic responsibility to be the best you can be and pass on that strength to the next generation. I want you to be that guy or gal that survives and lives on. As far as health and fitness goes, it's up to you to make it happen.

High-intensity Training

High-intensity training is the foundation of building full-body, general fitness. Without going into science, debating, and internet-troll-based-drama that usually comes with this topic, let me just tell you this: **HIIT produces fitness unlike anything else.** For those of you that have some fat to burn, high-intensity interval training (HIIT for short) is going to have the greatest effect on fat loss.

HIIT training looks like this: Perform exercise against the clock using weights, bodyweight, and functional movements. Using HIIT with a variety of movements and modalities is the secret sauce to developing elite fitness. "Variation" makes you well-rounded by targeting dormant muscles that don't get the exposure they need, while "functional" trains your body the way its meant to be trained: as a single unit. Combine the two and you have the best way of developing fitness.

After you build your foundation using constantly-varied, high-intensity training, you can focus on specific modalities for your goal or sport—like endurance training, rowing, running, swimming, strongman, Olympic weightlifting, powerlifting, etc.

Intensity

The professional athlete will train the same way to develop fitness as the soccer mom. The rules of fitness apply to everyone, regardless of individual goals or fitness level. The difference between two will be the weight and volume used. Obviously, the athlete will use more weight and more volume and need stricter recovery protocols while the soccer mom will get results using less weight and volume (and need less to maintain results).

Based on your goals and fitness level, you will establish what your baseline volume is through testing. Once you have established a baseline, you will constantly raise the bar (pun intended) as you get fitter by increasing volume and load. To keep making gains, you must keep taxing your body through training in a way that will bring supercompensation. Supercompensation is the process of your body over-adapting to training. It's how your body gets stronger, faster, and better. To continually reach this adaptive phase, you have to increase the stimulus your body receives after each successive recovery and growth period.

If you reach a point in your fitness that you are comfortable maintaining, you can focus on "maintenance." If you slip into maintenance mode, your body won't progress or regress, it will stay the same. This is where testing and tweaking your program comes into play.

Regardless of where you are at, you must constantly gauge how your body is responding to training so you can make adjustments up or down based on the feedback. For example, let's say you reach a point in your fitness that you are comfortable maintaining. You could then scale the volume back a bit to stay within that range. On the other hand, let's say you are still trying to make steady gains. In this case, you will keep challenging yourself by increasing weight, volume, and improved recovery protocols (sleep, nutrition) so you can keep progressing.

HIIT Workouts

Your HIIT workouts should be constantly varied using a wide array of modalities and movements. Most of your of workouts should be short and fast using high power outputs lasting under 10 minutes. Next you will train a mix of medium length workouts lasting 10-30 minutes at a slower pace, but not so slow as to be considered endurance. Finally, you will utilize endurance workouts lasting 30 minutes or longer. For most trainees, I suggest using these an average of once a week.

Intensity/time/volume:

The greatest misconception about exercise is thinking a longer workout is a better workout. This couldn't be further from the truth. The human body is a sensitive snowflake that needs just the right amount of the right inputs to produce a desired result. Training is good to a point, then overtraining sets in. Eating clean food is good to a point, then overeating sets in. Even sleep can be bad for you if you get too much of it too often (an extreme case).

For developing fitness, building strength and eliciting fat-loss, your body does best when you train as hard as you can for short periods of time. This is how you get results from high-intensity exercise: short, fast and hard. Contrary to popular belief, more training does not equal more results.

The longer you train, the more power output decreases and the less intense your workout becomes. It's an inverse relationship: more time = less intensity. Because the goal of HIIT training is to produce the highest power output possible, your results come training short workouts at your highest intensities.

As a general rule, half to two-thirds of your workouts should be in this highest-powered zone.

Because speed is the determining factor that separates training in the three metabolic pathways—phosphagen, glycolytic and oxidative—you want to stay cognizant of it at all times while you are training. During your HIIT workouts, speed and form are your primary concern. As you scale the speed back, you target different parts of your fitness. This is perfectly fine, and should be a part of your program, just make sure you aren't doing long conditioning workouts every session.

Too many trainees fall into the mindset trap of thinking that "more" and "longer" is better. You now see that short, intense, and hard is **better**. One-hour workouts that include a warm-up, strength work and 10-20 minutes of conditioning have proven to be the best dose for most people. This is the same template we use to train 350+ athletes in our box (and thousands that have come and gone).

Other Speeds

Like I said before, at least half (to two-thirds) of your conditioning workouts should be short and fast workouts lasting under 10 minutes on average. The rest of the time, you should be training at various speeds and modalities—especially your weaknesses. When you train high-intensity, you train all three metabolic pathways to varying degrees. When your train at a moderate-pace, you target the middle road of your fitness that utilizes a bit of power and a bit of endurance while less of the phosphagen pathway (highest powered). When you train endurance, you are operating in the oxidative pathway.

As you can see, by focusing on faster-to-moderately paced workouts, you target more of the metabolic energy systems. And this is, fundamentally, why you should reduce the amount of long-distance training in your program: because it does not provide enough benefit to your total fitness improvement for time spent compared to the shorter and more intense forms of exercise. Additionally, high-intensity training has been proven to increase performance in all the pathways, oxidative included.

The fitness formula is this: The shorter the workout, the more you can stay at your highest-powered intensities. The more power you produce, the more you improve total fitness. Thus, shorter, higher intensity workouts are more effective at developing total fitness.

A test you can do to understand the speed and power formula:

1. Complete a 100m sprint as hard as you can
2. In a few days: Run 1 mile as hard as you can
3. Next week: Run a 5k as fast as you can
4. Anytime: Walk 1 mile as fast as you can

Notice how each distance results in a different time and intensity? As distance and time increase, power output decreases proportionately—an inverse relationship. The goal for HIIT conditioning is to stay as close to the sprint and "all-out" 1-mile intensities as possible.

That said, other modalities all have their place in your program. In fact, neglecting them is detrimental to your fitness. They help make you a well-rounded athlete. Training long distances every so often will improve your fitness (I like once a week). Getting outdoors to jog, bike, walk or hike improves your fitness. Playing a sport with friends improves your fitness. And so on. I recommend doing each of these a couple times a week.

Now that we have covered how time correlates to fitness, I'll leave you with my recommendations for total fitness results-getting:

Make HIIT the focus of your conditioning. 3-4 times a week is best.

HIIT training is where the life-changing results are hidden, especially when you couple it with a weightlifting and nutrition program.

Because we are always pressed for time, I recommend HIIT training as the conditioning base for the majority of people. This will give you the best results in the least amount of time. With this as your base, you can strategically slip in the other forms of training based on your goals and weaknesses.

General Conditioning

Your results from conditioning (or anything in life) are <u>exactly</u> <u>equal</u> to the effort you put in. As you get better at training, you'll start to learn where your "redline" is. As you get more comfortable with your movement and training, you'll get better at pushing past this redline. This is what high-intensity in all about: to train at your highest levels for brief periods of time.

Training and Movement

Training is a skill-intensive endeavor that uses human movement, and there is generally a "wrong" way and a "right" way to move the human body. The best, and safest, way to utilize training is through the mastering of the fundamentals of movement. Fitness is an education and like anything else, it takes time to learn. Never forget this. If you're an ex-athlete just getting back into fitness, your abilities are going to be different than someone who has never touched a barbell in his or her life.

Your Body

High-intensity training and recovery are a happily married couple. If they get a divorce or separate, you'll have big problems. It's impossible to safely produce results without utilizing an intelligent recovery program consisting of nutrition, sleep, mobility, and "off" days. You can cause real damage to your health if you neglect these principles.

Overtraining is a real thing that is becoming more of a problem ever since the popularity of HIIT training hit the mainstream. There too many people hurting themselves because they aren't taking the time to learn the movements and account for the many variables that go into the whole that is fitness.

To avoid overtraining and injury, you must be patient with the process—you must kill the ego. Your body takes time to adapt to exercise, physically and neurologically. Rushing this process is just dumb. Gymnasts practice simple movements, like the handstand, for years. The same goes for Olympic Weightlifters that practice just 2 lifts for years. Don't assume you can start doing advanced movements with heavy loads right off the bat. No matter how fit you are, you have to progress through the process of skill and physical adaptation. You have to give it time.

A few recommendations:

- Get a foam roller and lacrosse ball and learn how to use each properly (myofascial release).
- Ask your coaches and utilize YouTube to learn which exercises can help you improve your weaknesses and how to work around injury.
- Start eating a clean Paleo or Primal diet.
- Avoid sugar and grains.
- Sleep at least 8 hours a night in a pitch-black room.
- Get sunlight daily.
- Eat Real Food in colorful variety.
- Legal disclaimer: Always consult your doctor before engaging in a training program.

The fundamentals of how to train your ass off with HIIT training:

1. Constantly increase intensity, volume, and loads as safely as possible.
2. Form first, speed second.
3. Always perform perfect reps. Don't sacrifice form for speed (like most do). You can have both if you train intelligently.
4. Vary your levels of intensity. Some days go to 75% of your redline, other days 99%, other days 50%, etc.
5. Think intervals: go hard for a few minutes then go slow for a brief period. Repeat.
6. Sprint.

Various modalities to train (get a coach):

- Sprint
- Row
- Bike
- Run (medium-long distance)
- Push/pull sleds, cars, anything heavy
- Move an external load
- Gymnastics
- Engage in natural movement
- Play sports

Low-intensity training

Low-intensity training is slow training. Remember, the body produces power via the mechanical power equation: force x distance x time = power.

As always, the key is balance. You must utilize many forms of conditioning. Low-intensity work is integral for recovery, skill development, and overall fitness improvement.

Kinds of low-intensity training:

* Any endurance based training
* Walking
* Mobility work
* Skill work
* Sled work
* Hiking
* Biking
* Swimming
* Jogging
* Climbing

Humans are made to move. Our hunter-gatherer ancestors walked an average of 13 miles a day. Compare that to the sedentary lifestyles of today—the average American now only walks 5,000 steps a day (and many walk much less). 5,000 might sound like a lot, but it's not, it's barely 2.5 miles. Our ancestors did 6 times that on any given day.

We are made to move often and at a slow-to-moderate pace. We are made to walk every day (you know, before the wheel was invented). Walking is great for recovery, improved digestion (especially after meals), and a great way to burn calories without infringing on your regular program. Go to NYC and you see a ton of reasonably skinny people walking around. They walk everywhere.

From now on, force yourself to take the longest route. This is your new mantra: move as often as possible. The more you move, the healthier you will be. This is a law of the human condition. Do everything you can to make yourself walk or move as often as possible.

Examples of moving:

- Taking a walk after meals
- Walking for 5, 10, or 30 minutes
- Parking at the end of parking lot
- Taking the stairs
- Walking your dog
- Take the longest route on purpose

Sports, Games, and Recreation

In addition to walking, you want to engage in as much physical activity as possible: sports, skill work, mobility, Yoga, hiking, walking, swimming, stretching, dancing, etc. By adopting a lifestyle that's full of movement, you get a bit closer to your goals every day without even thinking about it. Plus, it's more fun to lead an active lifestyle.

I'm a big fan of primal fitness: running, climbing, crawling, dragging, hanging, jumping, balancing, and moving in nature. Outdoor fitness is usually a missing link in most trainees program because so many get married to just going to the gym. The thing is...

> Your fitness is so much more than the gym.

Moving through terrain and obstacle helps target the weaknesses you pick-up from too much training in one or two modalities (like too much gym). Primal-style fitness and sports are the best way to fill in these gaps.

Our ancestors have been moving in nature for millions of years. Like the human diet, we have a "natural" training program that includes lots of walking, moderate amounts of running and sprinting, lifting and dragging heavy objects, and moving in nature in the form of swimming, climbing, crawling, and jumping. This kind of balanced fitness is what we are genetically predisposed to do based on what our ancestors did before us. You want to replicate this in your life as much as possible. This will help you avoid developing imbalances, improve your fitness, and make fitness fun and easier to maintain.

How To Get Primal

Go to parks, urban areas, hills, beaches, trees, the forest, a jungle, and move like your ancestors did. Make a game out of it, or set a clock for 45-minutes and just move. Be creative. Move. Then move some more.

Games and Sports

Humans have been playing and competing since the dawn of time. Sports are a great way to improve your fitness while also having fun. Sports often require short bursts of intense movements in many directions and this improves accuracy, balance, body control, hand-eye coordination, and footwork. Nothing can replicate the benefits of playing a sport like playing a sport.

How to play sports and games

Join an adult sports league, go to the park and play some basketball, get outside and chase your dog, play beach volleyball, etc. Aim for once a week or a few times a month—the more the better.

Examples of play include:
Running
Jumping
Balancing
Climbing
Swimming
Hand balancing

Places to play:
Park
Field
Forest
Jungle
Beach
Mountain
Hill

Tree
Playground
Trail

Sports and games:
Flag football
Dodgeball
Baseball
Kickball
Tennis
Obstacle courses/races
Kayaking
Surfing
Paddle-boarding
Etc.

Maintenance, Rest, Recovery

Most athletes love the training part of their fitness. I'm one of them: I love training. The thing is, **this is the easy part**. The hard part is spending time with the neglected stepchild of your results-getting efforts called: maintenance, recovery and nutrition.

It's not uncommon to find athletes that rush, shortchange or altogether skip certain parts of these much-needed protocols. Some even rush their warm-ups and cool-downs. Others avoid training their weaknesses. Most don't strength enough and work mobility. Some even convince themselves it's ok to eat "whatever" because they train so much. To make matters worse, athletes have a nasty habit of "cherry picking" workouts that complement their strengths while avoiding workouts that target their weaknesses. As a result, they further their imbalances and weaknesses.

The gym is an incredible tool for increasing functional fitness, but it has its limitations. You must spend time "out of the gym" as well.

Your "in-gym" and "on-field" training is only a piece of the total puzzle that is your results. Like training, maintenance and recovery require time and effort, and a healthy dose of each. Bodywork can be slow, boring, and even painful at times, but it isn't optional.

If you don't maintain your body, it will breakdown. Just like the car that isn't maintained. It's easy to fall into the trap of undervaluing maintenance and overvaluing training—in fact, most people do just that. That's a mistake.

Moving a bunch of weight or hitting a new PR might feel like more of an accomplishment than spending 30 minutes doing skill work but it's not always the case. There are times when training can actually negate your results and slide you backwards on the results scale. For some athletes, maintenance and the "outside of the gym" protocols are a hidden giant with the potential to explode their results.

The fact remains, you will hit more PRs, be safer doing so, and be able to train longer for the rest of your life if you add focused recovery and maintenance protocols to your program. Furthermore, know this: You will never reach your highest potential without proper rest, recovery, body maintenance, sleep and nutrition. Neglect them at your own peril.

How To Implement Maintenance and Recovery into Your Program

Before Training

Don't rush your warm-ups. They are integral to priming your body for the work ahead. Include mobility, skill work and some myofascial release (foam rolling) into your warm-ups.

Active Rest Days

Devote at least one day a week to active rest and recovery (some need more). The benefits of an active rest day cannot be overstated. Start doing them and watch your results skyrocket.

Maintenance work is composed of:

Flexibility: Use Kelly Starrett's book "The Supple Leopard" for recommendations
Weakness training: Take things you suck at and do lots and lots of reps of them at a slow pace.

Improving Weak Movement

Since your weaknesses often include muscular imbalances and flexibility issues, you will improve each when you improve your movement. Improving your movement consists of two principles—time and reps.

The time component has two parts:

- You must give yourself time to develop (be patient).
- You must perform movements as slowly as possible with perfect form.

The formula: Do lots and lots of reps as slowly and perfectly as possible with little to no weight.

For example, say you need to work on your back squat because you come off your heels and your depth is always debatable. This is what you do:

Grab a dowel and do super slow reps as perfectly as possible. Pick the speed up gradually as you improve. Go for sets of 20, 30, 50, or 100. Add small weight increments and repeat. After a couple hundred reps of hyper-conscious form, your squat will be noticeably better. Do this for a couple weeks and I guarantee you that your squat will no longer be an issue.

Repeat this formula with each weakness you have. On your active rest days, aim to perform 100-200 reps of various exercises you suck at—the more the better. You can also incorporate your weaknesses into your warm-ups.

Weakness Warm-ups:

Option 1:

- Weakness #1 for 3-5 sets of 12-15 reps
- Weakness #2 for 3-5 sets of 12-15 reps
- Weakness #3 for 3-5 sets of 12-15 reps

Option 2:

Perform 3x15 reps at a slow and deliberate pace:

- Air Squat
- Pistol
- Push-up
- Dip
- Strict pull-up
- Back squat with bar/dowel
- Overhead squat with bar/dowel

Randomize your warm-ups often and incorporate your weaknesses every chance you get. After a week of this, you will have completed hundreds of reps of your weakest movements. Soon after this, you will start seeing results.

Summary

If you start incorporating weakness techniques in conjunction with a balanced approach to your fitness, you will bust through plateaus and take your results to entirely new heights.

Here is an easy-to-remember template for an average training week:

-Lift weights and train conditioning three times a week
-Do something longer-distance at least once a week
-Train at least one maintenance session a week
-Get outdoors and move at least once a week
-Walk every day

A Hypothetical Training Week:

Monday: Squats followed by a sled-conditioning workout. 15 minutes of skill work at a moderate pace.
Tuesday: Play a pick-up basketball game. A 20-minute walk after dinner. A few sets of push-ups and stretching at home.

Wednesday: Bench press and upper body accessory work. Row 2500m at a slow-med page. Yoga for 15 minutes as a cool-down.

Thursday: Rest. Walk on the beach. Relax and smell the roses. This is known as an "off day."

Friday: Active recovery session and skill work for 1.5 hours in the gym. Legs sore from earlier in week so decide to work upper-body gymnastics (handstands, dips, rings). Ride bike for 20 minutes at a medium pace to speed up recovery.

Saturday: Lifting session of deadlift, Olympic weightlifting work, and GHD sit-ups. Beach volleyball, walk on beach, and enjoy a hard-earned cheat meal.

Sunday: Five-mile bike ride at a leisurely pace. Spend two hours prepping food for week. Complete 100 push-ups, sit-ups, and squats for time at home.

Above is an example of what my average training week looks like. Your average training week should be based on this template. How much more or less you do will come down to your preference, goals and fitness level.

My personal training strategy is based on taking a balanced approach to my fitness because my goals are longevity, improved fitness, and to look and feel good. I am not pursuing a sport or any performance-based goals. If I were, my training would reflect that. Since I'm only interested in health and looks right now, I utilize less in-the-gym volume and more outdoor and primal training. Also, for the last 13 years that I've been training my fitness, I've learned that my body does better with less gym-based volume and more outdoor, sport and Primal-style fitness. I also know I don't to do everyone else is doing—which is a lot of gym-based training. That said, I've learned what works for me and I stick to that. What works for you will be different. You have to figure it out for yourself (use this book as your guide).

For the rest of you that just want to be healthy and look good in the mirror, follow this schedule:

Train 2-3 times a week with adequate intensity, then throttle it back and do lower-intensity activities like those mentioned above. Get outdoors, move often, walk a lot, stretch and work mobility, eat a Real Food Paleo-based diet, enjoy friends and family, laugh a lot, be in the moment.

Great job... Now get to work!

Perfection is a fool's errand

Start small: Pick one or two techniques at a time and do them consistently until they **stick.** Keep building habit upon habit until you end up with your perfect program that is getting you the results you dream(ed) of.

This crazy thing we call health and fitness is all based on habits. Focus on consistency through habit, not perfection, and you'll get there. Keep going no matter what.

I just gave you the template for lifelong results... and it only cost you the price of this book! It's still going to be up to you to screw it up or make it work. Never forget that.

Remember, your brain is trying to keep you fat, lazy, and walking the path of least resistance. It's time to tell your brain to "shut the $#%@ up."

Eliminate the following words from your vocabulary: try, wish, hope, maybe, eventually, someday.

There is only DO or DO NOT.

There is no try. There is no tomorrow or later. Do something now or do it never. Now get doing!

Yours in Fitness,

-Colin Stuckert

About The Author

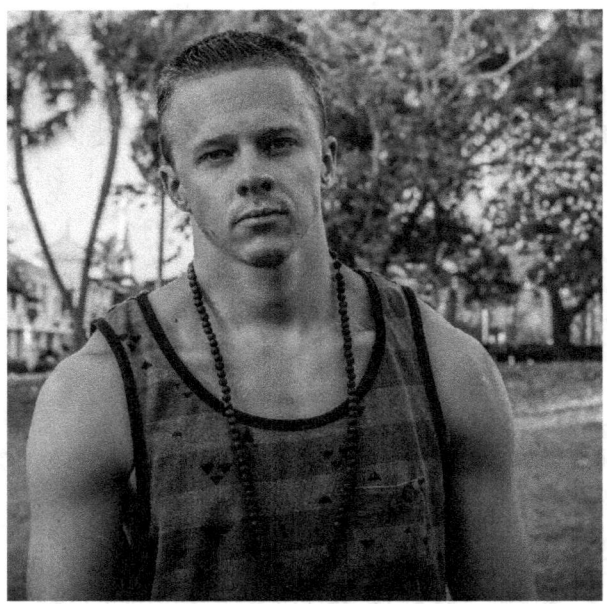

My name is Colin and I'm obsessed with personal development, food and fitness. Like Bruce Lee—my childhood idol—I believe in personal responsibility. What I get in my life is based on me. What you get in yours is based on you. Instead of complaining about the fairness of life and the good luck of others, I'd rather get working and make myself better.

"Time means a lot to me because you see I am also a learner and am often lost in the joy of forever developing."

-Bruce Lee

Of course, this isn't the easiest path. It's much easier to sit on the couch and make excuses. It's hard to do work every day... especially when it feels like you aren't moving anywhere... <u>but this is exactly what it takes</u>.

While others will quit after the grind sets in and their motivation wanes, I'll be plowing through (and I hope you will as well). And this is, in my opinion, what separates the winners from the losers, the wheat from the chaff, the cream to the top, the cat from the mouse, and so on.

What I do for a living

I started my first business in 2009: a juice and smoothie bar located inside a large corporate gym (ironic, I know). I started my second business 8 months later a few miles down the road—The Training Box—a group fitness and MMA gym. As I'm writing this, it's been 5 and a half years of learning, blood, sweat and tears, more learning, wasting money, making some back, being sued, spending (we call it "reinvestment" but sometimes I'm not so sure of the difference), plenty of stress, more learning, and now here.

I've worked *really* hard to grow my businesses to be as self-sufficient as possible. Recommend book on the subject: The E-Myth Revisited. Since I've been fortunate enough to attract a great group of people to work in my businesses, I now have the freedom of not having to work "in" my businesses, which allows me the time to pursue other passions (like writing). But it's still a lot of work. In fact, 95% (maybe more) of what it takes to run a business goes on behind "closed doors."

I went to college for a couple years but didn't do well. I stopping going right before speech class credit was due because I was afraid to speak in front of people (which is ironic considering I've had to use this very skill on a daily basis since I started teaching classes at our Box). *But such is life.* I never did well in school and I was always led to believe that I wasn't "smart" or that I would grow up to be a "loser." That's what they convince you of anyway.

When I discovered that you can work hard in your own business to determine your results, I was hooked. To me, personal development and success in business go hand-in-hand. Actually, I can't imagine being that good at business if you aren't good at making yourself better. It's the "always improving" mindset that succeeds. You have to face challenges head on and hustle to overcome them—and learn from the lessons so you are better next time.

Of course, there are many people that work hard, neglect their health, and still get results in certain areas of life. The thing is, I believe these poor souls could get more much greater results—plus all the benefits of being healthy—if they took a health-first approach. Personally, I'm utterly useless if I'm sick or tired. I just curl up in a little ball and my motivation to do anything disappears. This is why, for me, health always comes first. When I feel my best, I perform my best. When I improve myself, I get better at everything else. *This is my fundamental approach to life.*

I've meet many of these not so healthy yet uber-successful people over the years and their situations have always perplexed me. What's the point of having money if you can't enjoy it? Is it really worth working 80 hours a week just so you can watch the numbers in your bank account tick upwards? I don't get it.

If it were me, I would be traveling the world and getting into as much adventure as my success could finance. I would spearfish off the coast of Caribbean islands in a chartered boat, scuba dive in Australia near the great barrier reef, surf in Hawaii, climb mountains, experience new cuisines, meet interesting people from around the world, train with the Shaolin monks, learn urban survival from navy seals, and continually train to become the best version of myself possible and pursue causes that mattered to me. I guess everyone *is* different.

Food and Health

I'm obsessed with food and nutrition. I love to cook and I love to experience the best food I can find. I believe food is the most potent player in the health and longevity of a human being. I eat a Paleo and Primal style diet that consists of some dairy and no grains. I will have a "cheat" meal or two on the weekends, but for the most part I remain gluten-free. If I'm out of town and the occasion calls for it—like in Chicago for deep-dish pizza—I'll have grains. Other than that, I avoid grains because of their inflammatory effects on the body (and so should you).

If there were only one thing you could away from my work it would be **the importance of food.** You have to start eating real food if you want the best results, and/or to enjoy a long and healthy life. There is no way around it—no hack, tip, trick, or shortcut. Maybe when we invent nanotechnology that is able to reverse aging and cure disease, nutrition won't matter. But we don't have that technology, so until we do, food is the epicenter of human existence.

How to eat well:

- Avoid anything processed, refined, synthetic, artificial, etc.
- Cook your food at home as often so you can control the ingredients.
- Buy the highest-quality food you can find.
- Don't eat anything that isn't "real food."

My philosophy

I'm a practicing Stoic. In a nutshell, this means I base my decisions on only what is in my control—like my thoughts, emotions and actions—and I avoid wasting time on things out of my control—like other people, the weather, the past, the future. By taking this pragmatic approach to life, one sees how pointless things like anger, jealously, fear, and worry, actually are. Of course, as with everything, it takes practice. I regularly *catch* myself indulging in negative thoughts even though I've always been an optimist and I'm a consciously practicing Stoic.

I have yet to find a more practical way of living life. This would be my second most potent recommendation for you. Learn about Stoicism and other philosophy. Philosophy has the power to change your life. Here are some resources to help you:

Ryan Holiday Article on Tim Ferris Blog
The Art of Living: The Classical Manual on Virtue, Happiness, and Effectiveness

My health and fitness

I average 8-9% body fat year round. This fluctuates up or down depending if I'm traveling or have eating out a lot lately. I lift 3-4 days a week and target each main lift at least once (squat, deadlift, bench, press). I like to use gymnastics as "accessories" to the main lifts. I practice handstands and the basic holds/moves you see break dancers do (and no, I'm not a breaker... maybe one day). I incorporate some full-body functional training like sled work, farmer carries, and tire flips, at least once a week. I need to remind myself to sprint at least once a week. I just started swimming and am kicking myself for not utilizing this amazing form of exercise sooner.

Life

I'm passionate about life and aim to live each day to the fullest. Although this is tough as I often run into the problem of feeling like I'm not doing enough. This is a fault I struggle with. It's the byproduct of being too forward-minded. I tend to forget what *I've already done* and find myself focusing too much on *what I need to do.* I often have to remind myself to take breaks and spend time with friends and family.

I believe that relationships should be a constant pursuit in our lives. They are one of the most important things, if not thee most important. Unfortunately, I feel like so many of us let our relationships suffer when other things start monopolizing our time. And I think it's a grave mistake. Your work, school, project, or whatever should never take precedence over your relationships. Your relationships should always come first.

(This is as much a reminder for myself as it is my advice to you.)

My Work

Nowadays, I work with a couple clients in a consulting capacity to help them improve their web presence and marketing. I manage my two businesses and I spend the rest of my time writing, reading and researching topics of interest.

My ultimate dream is to make my full-time income from my writing. Since you are reading this, you have brought me one step closer to that dream. I don't take that lightly. **Thank you so very much.**

My other books are available on Amazon (here). I put out a ton of free content on my website AGymLife.com and the corresponding newsletter at GymLifeClub.com. If you want to get all the updates and exclusive list-only content, stop by and subscribe.

If you ever have any questions or need any help, please shoot me an email: ismynamecolin@gmail.com.

I'm here to help anyway I can. At the very least, feel free to share your comments by dropping me a quick note. It's always awesome to get words of encouragement from you guys that help me stay motivated. Amazon reviews also help (I print them out and put them on my wall)!

Yours in Fitness,

-Colin Stuckert

Resources

The following section includes quotes and links from the top experts in the world on all things fitness and training. I owe much of my education to them. You should definitely check them out. Also, there is something you should know about fitness:

There are many ways to skin a cat.

Some coaches produce world-class Olympic athletes using one style while others might use a completely different method and still send their athletes to compete for the gold. Keep that in mind the next time someone tells you this is the "only" or "best" way to train. Always test protocols out for yourself. Avoiding buying into any one fitness dogma, and never be closed-minded with your education. *Always be learning.*

Each human body will adapt differently to different forms of training. Some modalities will complement the things you are better at while others might target your weaknesses—and will probably get better results from the latter. Make sense?

I've said it before and I'll say it again: you must figure it out for yourself. You have the best *operational manual* to yourself. No one can tell you what your body is telling you. Listen to it.

Kelly Starrett:
http://www.mobilitywod.com/about/kellystarrett/

Author of Becoming a Supple Leopard and founder MobilityWod.com

Louie Simmons: http://www.westside-barbell.com

Powerlifting legend and Founder/owner of Westside Barbell and author of numerous books and articles

Mark Rippetoe: http://startingstrength.com

Author of Starting Strength

Mark Sisson: http://marksdailyapple.com

My go-to resource for all things ancestral-based health and nutrition. His site is all you need to learn everything you need to know about optimal health and nutrition.

Dave Asprey: http://www.bulletproofexec.com

The Bulletproof Exec and founder of the wildly successful Bulletproof Radio Podcast. His podcast is a must-listen.

Robb Wolf: http://robbwolf.com

My introduction to Paleo eating when I started out some 5 years ago. Robb is a pioneer of the Paleo movement and his podcast is great.

This short list comprises the majority of resources that have contributed to my education on these topics. You should buy their books, subscribe to their podcasts and newsletters, and support them anyway you can.

Tools

Fasting

Leangains.com
MarksDailyApple.com

Exercise

5/3/1 Program by Jim Wendler

Nutrition

Bulletproofexec.com
Robbwolf.com
MarksDailyApple.com

Tools

A Small Crockpot: This thing is AMAZING; consider getting 2 and loading them up each morning
Big Crockpot: great for bigger meals
Victorinox Chef Knives: Cheapest knives that still provide amazing results
Magic Bullet: I use this thing for my Bulletproof Coffee and protein shakes
Aero Press: Preferred way to brew coffee
French Press: 2nd preferred way to brew coffee. Also great for brewing loose tea
Cast-iron skillets: Last a lifetime, get an 8,10 and 12 inch)
Lacrosse ball: For trigger-point release

Food Ingredients
Bulletproof Coffee
MCT oil
Kerrygold Butter
Himalayan Sea Salt

Supplements

Ciltep By Natural Stacks
Performance Essentials stack by Natural Stacks
ZMA by Now Foods
Vitamin D by Now Foods
Vitamin C by Now Foods

Books

GymLifeCook.com: My book on cooking technique. Learn how to cook meals without the use of recipes by learning basic cooking technique you can use over and over.
GymLifeBook.com: My first book on all things fitness and health based on my work at agymlife.com
Tao of Jeet Kune Do: Bruce Lee is my childhood idol. This book is not just about fighting, it's pack-loaded with philosophy.
The Alchemist: International bestseller.
The Four-Hour Body: Tim Ferris fan. Check out his books.
The Richest Man in Babylon: Great book on money.
The Art of Living: The Classical Manual on Virtue, Happiness, and Effectiveness: This book can change your life. It had a role in changing mine.

Training Reference Guide
Get this in a PDF guide by going to
www.GymLifeClub.com

Here is an easy-to-remember template for your average training week:

Lift weights and train conditioning three times a week.
Do something longer-distance at least once a week.
Do at least one maintenance session a week.
Get outdoors and do random stuff at least once a week.
Walk every day.

A Hypothetical Training Week:

Monday: Squats followed by a sled-conditioning workout. 15 minutes of skill work at a moderate pace.
Tuesday: Play a pick-up basketball game. A 20-minute walk after dinner. A few sets of push-ups and stretching at home.
Wednesday: Bench press and upper body accessory work. Row 2500m at a slow-medium pace. Yoga for 15 minutes as a cool-down.
Thursday: Walk on the beach. Relax and smell the roses. This is known as a "rest day."
Friday: Active recovery session and skill work for 1.5 hours in the gym. Legs sore from earlier in week so decide to work upper-body gymnastics (handstands, dips, rings). Ride bike for 20-minutes at a medium pace to speed up recovery.
Saturday: Lifting session of deadlift, Olympic weightlifting work, and GHD sit-ups. Beach volleyball, walk on beach, and enjoy a hard-earned cheat meal.
Sunday: Five-mile bike ride at a leisurely pace. Spend two hours prepping food for week. Do 100 push-ups, sit-ups, and squats at home at a slow-medium pace.

The Training Session Format:

1) Body Temp Warm-up: Jog, Row, and move for 5

minutes until you break a sweat.

2) Dynamic Warm-up: Do movement based exercises at slow/light intensity to warm-up and loosen your joints.

3) Strength: Perform one or two main lifts a day to failure. Follow a program or stick with 5 sets of 5 at a weight you can barely complete on your last set.

4) Accessory Exercises: Choose 2-5 complimentary exercises and perform 8-15 reps over 3-5 sets. For example, do pistols (single-leg squats), weighted lunges, and glute-ham raises on your squat days, and do dips, floor presses and clapping push-ups on your chest/shoulder day.

5) Conditioning: Complete 5-25 minutes of high-intensity conditioning work.

6) Cool-down: Stretch, jog, walk, and keep moving for 5 minutes to let your body cool down gradually.

Set Schemes:
10 sets of 2 reps
8 sets of 4 reps
6 sets of 3 reps
5 sets of 5 reps
3 sets of 10
2 sets of 15+
1 set of 21+

WOD types:
AMRAP (as many rounds or reps as possible in X time) 5, 7, 9, 10, 12, 15, 20+ minutes

For Time: 2, 3, 4, 5+ rounds of 2, 3, 4, 5+ exercises for X reps (example= 5 rounds of 10 pull-ups, 10 pushups)

For Time: 100 reps of X

Tabata interval: any exercise or combination of exercises (4 min interval = 20 seconds work, 10 seconds rest until 4 minutes is complete)

10 50m sprints with rest between

In a pinch workouts:
Do a home/travel workout
1 mile run

5x 100m sprints
10x 50m sprints
For time: 100 pushups, 100 sit-ups, 100 air squats
For time: 50 push-ups, 50 air squats
For time: 100 burps (or as many as possible in 7 minutes)

Body Temp warm-up (3-5 minutes of light activity):
Row 500m
Run 500m
5 minutes jump rope
Incline walks
Bike

Dynamic Stretching Warm-up (5-7 minutes of movement-based stretching and moving)(mix these up in various reps and sets):
Squats
Lunges
Arm slaps
Arm circles
Wrist rolls
Neck rolls
Side bends
Runner's lunge
Push-ups
Sit-ups
Jumping jacks

Big Lifts for Strength (choose 1-2 for day):
Back Squat and variants: Front Squat, Overhead Squat, Box Squat
Deadlift and variants: sumo, stiff leg, Romanian,
Press and variants: push press, jerk, split jerk, seated
Bench Press and variants: floor press, DB press, incline, decline
Clean and variants: squat, power
Snatch and variants: squat, power

Common accessory exercises (choose 2-4 per strength exercise above as a compliment):
Squats
Deadlifts
Press
Jerk
Push-ups
Dips
Pull-ups
GHD sit-ups
Back extensions
Good mornings
Clean
Snatches
Kettle bell swings

Conditioning (5-20 minutes of various conditioning modalities):
5 mins - 10 mins - 12 mins - 15 mins - 20 mins - 30 mins - 60 minutes (sometimes)
Strongman
Circuits
Intervals (Tabata)
Swimming
Biking
Hiking
Play a sport

Cool-down (move for 3-5 minutes after workout):
Walking
Stretching
Skill work

Home/Travel WOD workouts requiring no equipment:
-For Time: 10 rounds of: 10 push-ups, 10 sit-ups, 10 squats
-For Time: 50 squats, 50 push-ups, 50 sit-ups
-For Time: 5 rounds of: Run 50m, 10 push-ups
-As many rounds as possible in 10 minutes of: 7 squats, 7

push-ups, 15 sit-ups

-Tabata squats - do as many squats as you can for 20 seconds, rest for 10. Repeat for 4 minutes

-For time: Run 1 mile, 100 Pull-ups, 200 Push-ups, 300 Squats, Run 1 mile

-4x 400M sprints - rest between

-10x 50m Sprint

-Run 1/2 mile 50 air squats – 3 rounds.

-10-9-8-7-6-5-4-3-2-1 sets of sit-ups and a 100 meter sprint between each set.

-Three rounds of: Run 800 meters, 50 Supermans, 50 Sit-ups

-10 push-ups, 10 sit ups, 10 squats – 10x rounds

-200 air squats for time

-3 rounds for time of: Sprint 200m, 25 push-ups

-Run 1 mile, lunging 30 steps every 1 minute.

-Handstand 30-60 second hold on wall and 20 air squats, 5 rounds.

-100 air squats for time

-100 burpees for time

-50 burpees for time

-For time: 4 rounds of: 10 broad jumps, 10 push ups, 10 sit ups

-10 air squats every 1 minute of your 1 mile run

-Run 1 mile for time

The Gym Life List of Usefulness

The Gym Life Essays: Improve Your Life Through Fitness, Food and Mindset: find it on Amazon

This is my first book (recently updated). Each chapter is an individual chapter with topics ranging from improving your fitness, 50 ways to lose weight, how to eat Paleo, and much more.

The Blog: www.aGymLife.com

I write about fitness, lifestyle, mindset, nutrition and health. New articles go up about once a week and I send an exclusive "only to my list" piece every Sunday.

The Gym Life Videos: www.GymLifeVideo.com

I make videos when I can find the time. There are a bunch of 20 Second Recipes videos. Check em out.

The Gym Life Podcast: iTunes

This is my new big project. Make sure you subscribe for all the updates. There are currently 14 episodes up. Feel free to listen and leave a review!

The Gym Life Library of Useful Stuff: http://agymlife.com/better/

This is a collection of bits of content ranging from books I recommend, quotes, tips, tricks, articles, videos, and anything else I find that I think is useful.

Disclaimer:

Consult a doctor before you engage in any exercise program.

The information provided in this book is designed to provide helpful information on the subjects discussed. This book is not meant to be used, nor should it be used, to diagnose or treat any medical condition. For diagnosis or treatment of any medical problem, consult your own physician. The publisher and author are not responsible for any specific health or allergy needs that may require medical supervision and are not liable for any damages or negative consequences from any treatment, action, application or preparation, to any person reading or following the information in this book. References are provided for informational purposes only and do not constitute endorsement of any websites or other sources. Readers should be aware that the websites listed in this book may change.

This book is designed to provide information and motivation to our readers. It is sold with the understanding that the publisher is not engaged to render any type of psychological, legal, or any other kind of professional advice. The content of each article is the sole expression and opinion of its author, and not necessarily that of the publisher. No warranties or guarantees are expressed or implied by the publisher's choice to include any of the content in this volume. Neither the publisher nor the individual author(s) shall be liable for any physical, psychological, emotional, financial, or commercial damages, including, but not limited to, special, incidental, consequential or other damages. Our views and rights are the same: You are responsible for your own choices, actions, and results.

www.ingramcontent.com/pod-product-compliance
Lightning Source LLC
Chambersburg PA
CBHW070121290526
45789CB00005B/2097